2022

Andrew Aldred

chipmunkapublishing
the mental health publisher

Published by
Chipmunkapublishing
United Kingdom

http://www.chipmunkapublishing.com

Copyright © Andrew Aldred 2022

ISBN   978-1-78382-6278

Dedication

To my darling Jane.

Andrew Aldred

Have You Had Enough

I would like to ask Boris Johnson where it will all end?
We are getting stories about Peppa Pig during speeches about industry
Is that all there is in your head when you talk to the unions?
Like Winston Churchill and Margaret Thatcher, you will go eventually
Whether it is because of your own volition or the pack of wolves that surrounds you
All too many people want to make you responsible for their own misfortune
Margaret Thatcher resigned, and Winston Churchill got voted out
If you do not pull yourself together quickly you will be next
Everybody has a breaking point and a sell by date, and you are no different
You have carried the country through a particularly difficult few years
Maybe the time when somebody else can step up to the plate is coming
You have done your best but when will everybody say they have had enough?

Get the Booster

There are riots throughout Europe
People not wanting the vaccine
It does not matter how the virus has come about
An act of revenge by mother nature
Something created in a government chemical laboratory
Or just an accident in a Chinese market
It is everywhere and has been for two years
They are predicting many deaths this winter
You can shout all you want about big brother
Sabotaging humans and killing everyone
But if I were you, I would get the booster
If you want to survive a winter where many will die

Give them Jobs

These are the people fit to flee
From the tyranny in their own country
They are determined to find a better life
And they cross the channel and risk their life
They have all got to fit in somewhere
Whether its France or Germany or over here
We ought to take our quota of refugees
As ought the people in other European countries
These people are generally fit to work
Or they would not have made it over here
They ought to be allowed to work
And put their shattered lives together
I am sure we could find a better way
Then people dying in dinghies every day
I do not want to hear of people drowning on the news
It is time the politicians found some common ground
And sorted this humanitarian crisis out

Fahan

The parcel for my latest set of books got delivered recently
The only thing wrong was it got delivered to somebody called
Fahan
I set about tracking it down knowing Fahan means "boy" in Asian
But after asking the Asian neighbors and the local shop I drew a
blank
I looked up Fahan again and found it was a place in County
Donegal in Ireland
Some Irish folks had recently cleaned my drive, but I could not
trace them
And the last thing I want is a barney with an Irish family from
Salford
All I can do is wait for the books to be reprinted and sent again
I am old and tired, nearly fifty-six and I want a peaceful Christmas

Going Bananas

The whole world is going crazy at the moment
It's not just Boris Johnson, its everyone I know
People are so short tempered these days
Half of Farnworth is outside ASDA drinking
Begging for money, and not all of them are genuine
The weather has turned cold and there has been another storm
My lager consumption is creeping up again, and I am so tired
Thirty years of heart problems and mental illness, and cancer
Are taking their toll on me and what I am capable of
I guess I will just sit in and quietly go crazy
And hope the rest of the world will keep turning without me
I really wish I could rest but life still goes on

Beasts

I keep the beast in myself under control
Other people unfortunately are not able to
I sleep mostly in a locked room at night
Unless I have a beer and sleep on the couch
I have to watch myself if I am away from home
Outwardly I have an easy time and get on with my life
But nearly forty years of confusion and illness
Since I left the army at the age of twenty
Have left me mentally and physically shattered
I try to get on and not to fall behind
In a world that is more and more hostile
Life does not always get easier as you grow older
The beast in myself died a long time ago
But in other people it is still alive and strong
There is no longer any fear, but I have to be careful
In this modern society there are beasts everywhere

Sacrificed

The sad case of a boy named Arthur
Came on television and left us all outraged
A boy with multiple bruises trapped in a situation
We question the police and the social services
Who seem to have been shut out by the parents?
The grandma and uncle tried to help
But the parents seemed determined to carry on
With systematic abuse and cruelty
You wonder what the world is coming to
The parents were to blame, and Arthur was the sacrifice

Andrew Aldred

Work Until You are Ninety

I saw a young man on TV today
Who wants to work until he is dead?
Well good luck with that, my son
We are all ready to collapse at fifty-five
It is ok for you to preach when you are twenty-one
What about the rest of us, do we not count?
People need to have a choice but there is none
They will find a use for you until you pass away
You will be doing something until you are ninety
If you manage to last that long, whatever it is?

Who will replace Them?

There have been endless accusations of sleaze
About Boris Johnson and the Tory party
But is Keir Starmer really any better?
I think he knows in his heart he is not
Or he would have seized the opportunity by now
If he really wanted to rule, he would be doing it
But he would rather be a heckler for his own reasons
The Tories have got some good policies and get things done
It is ok complaining, but would things be better under Labour?
The opportunity to have a Labour government is coming
But what ideas do they really have and how different are they?
It seems to me they are happy to be an opposition party

Big Narstie

I watched your show on TV the other day
And all it seemed to do was condone illegal drugs
You had the model who offered LSD to her friends
The Muslim comedian who was so obviously off his head
A black politician who wanted to support the Labour party
And seemed more concerned about lies than politics
And Digga D the rapper who seemed the best of the bunch
And you and your cohort who had to hold it all together
But you all seemed to be off your heads on drugs
Is this a sad reflection on society or on you?
Not all black people rely on drugs to be interesting
A lot of them have some genuine talent at something
You need to do better if you want me to watch your show

Genetically Modified

Not all people are created the same
A lot of us have defects at birth
Some of us are grown to be a certain way
A lot of it seems to be manipulated with drugs
We seem to want to be part of a genetic experiment
I want no part of this and never have done
People will lead you up the garden path
You will be ok if you can just be yourself
Dump the silly bastards who want to change you
Know yourself, that you are alright, and you will be
What we are born with is hard enough with no modifications

The Anti-Hero

I am the anti-hero but at least I am alive
I do not stand out, but I am here
I would tell you my story, but it is better not known
I have survived all sorts of shit and continue to
And if you have any sense, you will leave me alone
At every death there is an inquest and an autopsy
I am nothing like Andy McNab or Ant Middleton
My details are well hidden on an army database
I am so deep in the system you cannot see
I have had many opportunities to die but have always refused

I will be Getting On

I guess I will carry on with my life as long as I can
And I guess that is up to everyone else and not me
I will do what you ask me too as far as I am able
And if I default on anything do not blame me
I have always done my best and will continue to
I love my girlfriend and I will try for my family
But if I am not who you expected do not blame me
We will have another Christmas largely on our own
We will probably see her mother on Christmas day
Everyone else will be getting on with their arrangements
The world will turn, and God will be in his heaven
I need to get on with my life and not bother
We are all expendable and I am no different to anybody else

Do as I say and not as I do

It is a sad reflection of the times
When the Tory party does what the hell it wants
While the rest of us try to get on with our lives
It was always like this when I was in the army
Our superiors always carried on like they were gods
And expected us to put up with their shit
But eventually people get tired of the status quo
Unfortunately, we all have to play by our own rules
Because that is the only way we will survive intact
We have had officials in China with a tennis scandal
The Royal family have had their issues with America
And it cannot all be glossed over and covered up
We should all be upholding the rules from the bottom up
Do as I say and not as I do does not work any more

Been Around the Block

I have been everywhere at least once
I do not need to go there again
I learned what I could about the army
The prison system, education and work
I have a mental illness that is very real
The only place that can help me is the hospital
Or the local GP if they can see me
I can do everything for myself now
I have a house, a car, and they are all mine
I really need some time on my own now
It will not be much of a Christmas for me
I will get better and face the world again
I am a small cog in a big machine
I am worn out and now it is time to replace me
I have always been free in my mind if nowhere else

The Pedophile Prince

I am so sick of this public witch hunt
Prince Andrew and Ghislane Maxwell should have known better
All this ugly news revolves around is money
The girls they employed as escorts were not innocent
Everyone knew what they were engaging in and what they were doing
And I hope they are all satisfied with the outcome of this case
People forget the Prince's Trust and that Andrew is a war hero
Ghislane Maxwell has been treated like an animal in prison
All that for a few girls with bad reputations chasing money
Jeffrey Epstein was guilty and has committed suicide
When and where is this sad and pathetic story going to end?

Slowly Going Crazy

I have been slowly going crazy for many months now
My paranoia at night has been increasing
My alcohol consumption has been incrementing slowly
I have been busy doing everything for myself and my girlfriend
I have been having heart problems with the stress of it all
And I desperately need to press the reset button to survive
I decided to bite the bullet and go it alone before Christmas
She sent me a Christmas card and we got back together
I told her my problems and she understood to a level
We had a good Christmas although I did not sleep over
I will be sleeping over tomorrow, and I hope it goes well
We will be together on Friday when we see our grandson
Life has never been easy for two physically and mentally disabled
people
But we have been through hell and high water many times and
survived

Sending the Wrong Message

Donald Trump supporters did their insurrection a year ago today
And everyone thinks it was just another riot
People think they can do what the hell they want and get away
with it
What is next? Will they storm the White House?
Sooner or later a lot of people are going to get shot
And the stupid thing is they will wonder why?
You can only bend the rules so far before things break down
It has happened in Kazakhstan over petrol prices
They will bring the military in if they cannot do anything else
Donald Trump was a highly irresponsible president
He should have faced a jail sentence but never did
They are making examples out of people like George Floyd every
day
But the real criminals are let off and rewarded
We are a society full of hypocrisy and double standards
The people in charge play us for fools all our lives

Unfit to Govern

We have heard it all now and let's hope there is no more
Boris Johnson and a hundred conservatives at a garden party
At the height of the pandemic when the country was in lockdown
Everyone is disgusted and rightly so. This was a betrayal
This arrogant and hypocritical man has to be thrown out of office
Most people have followed the rules at huge personal expense
Not able to comfort the dying and unable to see relatives
But how different it is for the people in charge, and it should not
be
Johnson and his party should have followed the rules to the letter
If they could not, they have shown themselves unfit to govern
We are all sick of the double standards and sleaze of this
government
They had better get somebody in who will practice what they
preach
And that is a tall order for people who think they are above us

Andrew Aldred

The Coulson Four

They were let off just the other day
The people who had taken down the statue
The black mayor did nothing to remove it
And endless petitions got continually ignored
A set of middle-class white kids tore it down
And they did not even serve a prison sentence
Because they had the right haircuts and clothes
If they were black or lower class, it would be different
But at the end of the day, they did us all a favour

Time to Go

They are saying they want the enquiry
To tell them what is right and what is wrong
God knows why because I certainly do not
There has been party after party for two years
And the man in charge has turned a blind eye
While the rest of us have suffered their rules
Boris does not have a leg to stand on, but we still wait
For yet more details of conservative double standards
There is corruption on a grand scale with this government
I am tired of waiting. It is time they went

Novak Djokovic

Novak Djokovic has no respect for the people of Australia
He will not get the injection and follow the rules
He expects the whole world to bow down to him
He thinks tennis needs him more than he needs tennis
But that is not the case and I hope he gets excluded
He has been instrumental in creating his problems
He has upset a lot of people who have had the vaccine
And expected to go there without it and get applauded
He is a great tennis player, but he is not living in the real world
He needs to get vaccinated and realize he will be no worse off

Let it Roll
The trial of Prince Andrew is going ahead
There is no way to wriggle out of it
He has been stripped of military and Royal rank
And left to fight the court case on his own
Virginia Giuffre is going to take him to the cleaners
And he will end up a sad and broken man
Whether he spends time in prison or not
The mighty fall with an almighty crash
The prince looks as guilty as hell in recent photographs
An ugly and infuriated man who will not back down
The Queen has abandoned him and that is a bad sign
The courts are going ahead, and it will be a catastrophe

Andrew Aldred

Bad Apps

They want you to load this and then load that
And all the while it takes memory on your phone
Which has everything you wanted on it anyway
You end up with multiple boosters and cleaners
When all you needed was what you got with the phone
I have recently purged my phone of all unwanted apps
And lo and behold it has freed up a lot of memory
They all want you to buy into their advertising
And it is such a waste of time for a fifty-six-year-old man
I am not interested in tik Tok or even the bloody co-op
If you want your phone to last get rid of the bad apps

Tonearm Wires

My turntable has only been working on one channel recently
I took it in for repair, but he did not want the job
And told me it was ok, and I was worried about nothing
So, I bit the bullet and sorted it out myself
I took the old wires and the tonearm to pieces
Put in some new wires and rebuilt the tonearm
Then I soldered it and checked for errors
Eventually I thought I had got it sorted out
And put it back together for the last time
This turntable cost six hundred quid in the nineties
But all my efforts eventually came to nothing
I got rid of the turntable and traded my other one in
I cannot fix everything, and I have to cut my losses

Not Giving it Away

You can knock on my door asking for money
But I do not have anything to give away
You are not a charity unless I am mistaken
If I give my money away it is no good to me
If you do something for me, it is a different story
And I will reach my hand in my shallow pockets
And hand over what you want for your services
I have little enough, and I am not giving it away

False Economy

It is all very well buying second hand everything
But there is always a reason someone has got rid of it
You end up paying for everything twice or three times
When if you bought new you would only pay once
There is nothing worth buying in the charity shops
Someone has always got the good stuff before you
It is all very well trying to make do and mend
But everybody knows secondhand goods do not last

Taking back What is Theirs?

Russia invaded the Crimean Peninsula in 2014
And now they are pressing on to take Ukraine
They are territories that used to be Russian but defected
Europe depends on Russia for a lot of its oil and gas
I know Russia is an aggressive state under Vladimir Putin
But is one state worth starting the third world war?
Ukraine is divided between nationalists and pro-Russian people
What can we do apart from get our own nationals out?
Joe Biden and Boris Johnson come out with a lot of trash talk
But Putin only has to blink an eye and the territory is lost
And if we want Russia's oil and gas we had better not look
And let them get on with restoring the Russian empire
I want to be able to drive my car and keep warm this winter
And the rising cost of fuel is terrifying for many people
If you are driving a car, you do not want to run head on into a lorry
And that is exactly what will happen if we decide to take Russia on

Cassette Crazy

I noticed cassette tapes were three times their normal price
And I have realized it is something to do with supply chains
A week later cassette tapes and decks were a normal price again
I have a large collection of pre-recorded cassette tapes
And I have bought a cassette deck and numerous cassette tapes
In the hope the shortage of supply does not catch me out again
I have invested a lot of money in this form of electronic media
I have gone cassette crazy, and I hope this medium does not die

Andrew Aldred

War With Russia

Is it really a good idea to be so vocal against Russia?
While China is standing dormant in the background
We had better remember we are dependent on them for oil and gas
And realize we are no longer in the old days of colonialism
Where we could take anyone on and beat them in a war
Russia has the biggest nuclear arsenal in the world
When I was in Germany, we were given two minutes to live
In the event of a Russian invasion and Europe would fall
Within a week they would have invaded the United Kingdom
Ukraine is divided as to whether it wants to be Russian or
independent
There is very little support for us from the rest of Europe
We might be the only nuclear state to stand against Russia
The Americans are a safe distance away and do not have to care
The entire world has just come out of a pandemic, and we are
struggling
I am sure shouting our mouths off will do not good
A war with Russia is one we will not win

Will Sanctions be Enough?

The British and the Americans are targeting Russian banks
Billionaires, the elite and the super-rich and their families
The Germans have called a halt to the gas pipeline from Russia
It looks like the Americans are taking things seriously this time
And not turning away as we did with Georgia and Crimea
But how crazy is Putin and what allies has he got?
Is the gas deal with China backed up in any way?
It is very important things are allowed to de-escalate
And Russia is frustrated in its attempt to overthrow Ukraine
Putin has a gigantic reserve of money to draw on
It will be a while before Russia feels the pinch of the sanctions
The West has got to stand in a united front against this man
And somehow unpick what he is doing and reverse it
Everything will become clear, and we will know what we face
NATO is standing as a unit against the Russian state
And if any members get attacked, we will all pitch in
We have to turn things against Putin and the Russian parliament
It will take more than sanctions to make Russia listen

God Bless Ukraine

The Ukrainians are having to stand largely on their own
With limited help from Europe and other nations
Against the might of a heavily armed Russian army
I do not think Russia wants a war with the West
They thought Ukraine would fall easily and welcome them in
But that is not the case, and it is not going to be
We are concentrating on drawing Russian wealth from foreign
banks
Sending arms and ammunition to the war zone
Nuclear war has been avoided and I hope it will be
But we are all going to be left with bills to pay
Oil, gas and everything else will be more expensive
The world did not need this conflict happening
God bless Ukraine for standing up and I hope we would be as
brave
We can help them, but we cannot declare war on Russia
God knows this conflict is better off being contained
I am so sorry this situation has happened. Bring back peace in
Europe.

Is Putin Crazy?

President Macron of France spoke to President Putin yesterday
And he said that Putin's version of reality does not tally with us
We have the invasion of a sovereign country and the threat of
nuclear war
And we are reduced to creating sanctions and providing help
For a nation in Europe that is getting obliterated by its neighbor
Putin is crazy but he knows exactly what he is doing
He talks about Nazism in Ukraine and the threat of nuclear
weapons
And we did the same in the conflict with Saddam Hussein's Iraq
But that has been forgotten and is there any truth in Putin's
claims?
He has vowed to press on until he has taken Ukraine
The rest of the world does not see eye to eye with him
Either we are all getting it wrong, or President Putin is
He is a rogue dictator with a large nuclear arsenal
We do not know what his agenda is, and I fear the worst

Andrew Aldred

A Sad Day for Europe

An army of Russian conscripts march forward
Attacking their neighbors and fellow countrymen
They did not bargain on having any resistance
From a state they thought they were liberating
The rest of Europe has to watch on in horror
Because of the very real threat of nuclear war
We are having to bow down to a dictator
Because of his nuclear weapons and firepower
Everybody is tired and how long will it go on for?
A humanitarian crisis and a million refugees
Vladimir Putin refuses to even call it a war
Russians are protesting and the jails are full of them
Sports and media have taken sides in this conflict
Russia cannot even sell oil and gas to Europe
We do not want anything to do with Putin's Russia
Russia and the rest of Europe are entrenched in two sides
This is a sad day for Europe and will take years to put right

Who is Going to Dare Win This War?

The Russians are marching on and threatening nuclear strikes
We are talking about giving Ukraine Polish aircraft
Ukraine is asking us to enforce a no-fly zone across its country
There is a mass exodus and those left are fighting for their lives
Civilians are being shot down by the Russian artillery
We are applying sanctions but is that all we can do.
How far can we defy Russia without it accelerating into war?
Sometimes I think we ought to test the Russian dictator's mettle
He says he can obliterate all NATO countries and America
Does he not realize we can also do him significant damage?
When are we going to step up to the plate?
When is he going to back down and send his troops home?
Sometimes I think it is going to take a reckless and dangerous act
To make a terrorist dictator see what lies ahead
We can only skirt around issues for so long before we commit
ourselves

Desperate

I saw the Ukrainian president on TV today
And there was a change of tone in what he was saying
I saw a man who was drowning in desperation
Who wanted the West to act and act quickly
A million refugees have gone to Poland
Anyone with any sense should be leaving Ukraine
The Russians are going to blow Ukraine to bits
Vladimir Putin is incensed by the actions of the West
We have done everything we can apart from declare war
Are Ukraine and its president going to have to be martyrs?
The resistance seems to have made a bad situation worse
How is this nightmare situation going to play out?
What Putin has done will become public knowledge in Russia
And that could bring about his downfall
The West stands firm and united, but we have sacrificed Ukraine
Almost all of the Russian army is in convoys around Kyiv
The entire situation is a mess, and nothing has gone to plan
For Ukraine or Russia and we watch and wait in the shadows
This is a desperate situation that is way out of hand
And how anybody is going to put it right is beyond me

Nicola Sturgeon's Nonsense

I am so sick of hearing this woman's point of view
She does not want nuclear armaments in Scotland
She is not aware that while we have nuclear missiles
We still have a voice against Russia and other nuclear states
And without nuclear armaments we are impotent and left open
To be trampled on, ignored and even invaded
Other countries do not give a shit about nuclear disarmament
They want to get ahead and get their voices heard
Nicola Sturgeon wants everything her own way
But she is not prepared to sacrifice anything
She wants England to have nuclear weapons and defend her
And she chooses a moment when Europe is in crisis
To parade her silly point of view to the world
While we are all living under the threat of nuclear war
Sorry, Nicola, but you could not run a kid's tea party
Never mind Scotland, look in the mirror today
And ask yourself whether you are living in the real world?

Andrew Aldred

Need for Dialogue

Russia and America have been insulting each other
The states nearest to Ukraine have been trying to sort things out
Russia is failing in its invasion of Ukraine
But the whole country needs rebuilding and repair
There has been talk of a ceasefire and compromise
But the Ukrainians are justifiably angry, and Russia will not relent
This war has turned brother against brother and father against son
It has gone far enough and needs to be sorted out
Ukraine cannot join NATO and will never be allowed to
It needs to be a neutral country between Russia and the west
There are some areas of Ukraine that would rather be Russian
Why the fuck did it come to the brink of nuclear war?
The politicians need to get around a table and sort this out
We all need to talk to each other and stop scoring points
People are dying every day and millions have been displaced
Everybody had better shoulder the blame and start getting on
There is a desperate need for dialogue in Ukraine right now

Pray for Peace

We watch in horror every day
As the war continues and unfolds
We donate to charities for Ukraine
And watch the concert on television
We see Russia say one thing and do another
Putin is going to cut off our gas supplies
His army is losing and being turned back
But when will it all be over?
Everyone is praying for peace and an end
To this abhorrent war on our doorstep
We stand united with Ukraine in the West
And we hope China will stand with us
Against Russia on this very important issue
We watch and pray every day for peace
Knowing we will be next if it gets out of control

Religious Heresy

There are a lot of practices in religion
That go against the ethics of love and harmony
They show the gay conversion ceremonies today
The government has said it will reverse the law
The Queen has promised she will do the same
Yet they all do nothing and let things carry on
There is genital mutilation and circumcision
That hardly gets mentioned these days
There is the Jihad and the prophet of war
And to any right minded and peace-loving person
It should be so much hocussed pocus and bullshit
There are the endless admissions of child abuse
Coming to light thirty or forty years later
And still people want to practice religion
I do not agree with any of these customs
And I exercise my right not to go to church
Religion is the highest level of hypocrisy
And the church is a very rich institution
You can buy into it. It is all about money
As well as power, abuse and control
If anyone needs religion, I certainly do not
I believe in a God that is kind, loving and humane

Outdated and Disintegrating

The Royal family hark back to a bygone era
When they were the godhead of the country and an almighty
institution
You look around and sometimes see that is not the case
The Queen is ninety-five and nearing the end of her life
There has been the death of Diana and the excommunication of
Harry
The misfortune of Prince Andrew and Virginia Giuffre
And somehow, we are supposed to buy into all of this
Commonwealth countries are leaving left, right and center
We desperately want somebody to get behind and lead us forward
All we have is Charles and Camilla and William and Kate
Do we really need a Royal family, or has it had its day?
Will it die with the Queen who has held it together for so long?
The days of colonialism are long gone, and people see through
them
Perhaps it is time the monarchy stepped down and we became a
Republic

Joe Biden is Right

Joe Biden said the Russian people should replace Putin
Other heads of state would not go so far
But Putin has been made to look cheap by us
He is failing in his invasion of Ukraine, and we will not trade with
him
His generals lie to him, and his soldiers do not believe in him
He is the most out of touch man in the whole of Europe
And he is leading the premier nuclear-powered nation
We hope his own people will deal accordingly with him
Because if they do not it will spell disaster for all of us

Run Off Your Feet

You have got a great deal of responsibility
Our parents are in care and need attention
You have moved into their house with your girlfriend
And you need to save some money to get your own
There are a million things to transport from her house
And a million things to sift through and get rid of
You are working five days a week at your job
And you hardly get any relaxation on your days off
I appreciate what you are doing and hope you see it through
To a time when you are married and with your own house
And our parents can go to their graves taken good care of
I wish I could help you more, but my partner needs me
We have our own property and her mother's to look after
And she needs help and transport to look after her family
I hope you can get yourself sorted out and in a good situation
But until then you are probably going to be run off your feet

Shooting Their Mouths Off

My girlfriend watches Jeremy Vine and the extra program
And I must admit I do when I am at her house
And it seems to be people who do not know what they are talking
about
Voicing their often-ridiculous opinions and having an argument
I know they probably cannot get the guests to do anything better
But the bullshit people talk and how self-important they are
Makes me wonder what the hell I am doing watching it
Empty vessels make most noise and Jeremy Vine is full of them
Shooting their mouths off on national TV and getting paid for it

A Summer of Gardening

I have planted my potatoes, my onions and some greens
And I will wait for them to grow in my pots and trays
The grass is going to need cutting at my house and her mother's
I cut down some trees over there last winter
And the council carried away the waste in the green bins
All I will have to pay for is my tall hedge to be cut
I am too old to go up there and do it myself now
The war in Ukraine is going to drag on and prices will rise
I will do what I can to save some money and feed us
A summer of gardening seems to be the best solution to my
problems

Oldies but Goodies

I spend my spare money on rock and roll
Records and CDs from my youth and more recent stuff
It is an insurance policy in a world of increasing prices
All these relics appreciate in value as they grow older
And they do not always get re-released as artists die off
If I am down to my last bean, I can always sell them on eBay
I only collect what I like, and I do listen to them all
I replace CD cases and the inner sleeves from the records
And try to make sure everything I keep is in good condition
Knowing someday it will be worth something to who is left

Killing Eve

I have been watching Killing Eve on BBC iPlayer with my
girlfriend
It is the most bizarre series and very entertaining
It centers around the key character, an assassin called Villanelle
Who is instructed to travel around murdering people
For a secret society of twelve chosen people
Who give her the jobs, which she carries out in outrageous fashion
And how on earth she remains at large is beyond me
And Eve is some sort of MI6 agent on Villanelle's trail
And there is some weird, kinky lesbian thing between them
Then there is Constantin, his associates and the KGB
It is the strangest thing I have seen on television for awhile

A Softer Ride

I need people to be gentle with me as I grow older
I do not wish to suffer further from the illness I have
I have not got what it takes to work for a living again
And I cannot do everything I used to for people
My asthma, arthritis and heart problems have got worse
I recovered from cancer, and I do not want it again
I could really do with everything going right for me for a change
Can things be alright for awhile and can I have a softer ride?

More War Crimes

There have been multiple war crimes in the Ukrainian conflict
Brutal killings of children and civilians, and multiple rapes
As humanity sinks well below what it should be once again
And the crimes of Bosnia are committed again in a different
country
We have a strict code of conduct in the British military
And I would like to think it is held sacred and enforced
It did not keep Tony Blair from sending soldiers to Iraq
Over trumped-up ideas of weapons of mass destruction
We turned Afghanistan upside down because of the Twin Towers
Only to let the people who believed in us down
I thought the Falklands was a just war, but there were oilfields
And not all of the people on the Island cared about being British
War is a dirty business without the atrocities that go with it
I hope Russian perpetrators are held responsible and face justice

Pairing Off

Most people in our family have a partner these days
Jane's daughter has found a man and I hope it lasts
They are travelling to Canada on a working holiday
My brother has teamed up with a woman he previously knew
She got in touch with him after a few years apart
There are Jane and me, Jane's niece and her partner
My mother and father, and Jane's sister and brother-in-law
In fact, there are not many people that have not paired off
I hope we can all keep it together and get on
And remain settled and happy for many years to come